Alternative Medicine:
20 Proven Hacks How to Make & Use Homemade Remedies to Prevent and Heal Illnesses

The information herein is offered for informational purposes solely, and is universal as so. The presentation of the information is without contract or any type of guarantee assurance.

The trademarks that are used are without any consent, and the publication of the trademark is without permission or backing by the trademark owner. All trademarks and brands within this book are for clarifying purposes only and are the owned by the owners themselves, not affiliated with this document.

Table of content

Introduction

Home remedies include using various vegetable, spices, drinks and many natural things like these to treat illnesses or even prevent them but have no scientific basis and evidences. Home remedies are becoming more and more popular as the modern medicine is getting more and more expensive and has more side effects than curing effects while home remedies might or might not have properties of medicine for the illness at the hand but they also don't have any side effects.

As herbs don't have any kind of side effects, they are not expensive and easily accessible and have no chemicals, there use is becoming more and more common but herbs effectiveness is not a news, old folks have been using herbs from the ancient times. They would grow different kind of herbs in their garden and then whenever needed, these herbs would be used by them to cure or prevent illnesses. From simple flu to boosting child's immune system, treating hair fall and acne, treating pains and aches or even treating burns and cuts.

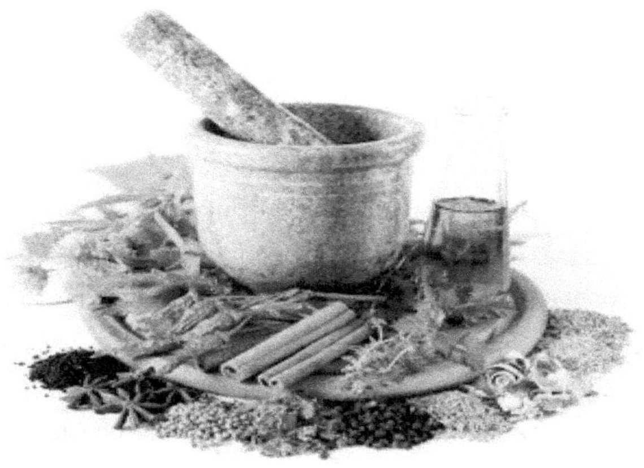

Home remedies that has been used for centuries and by almost everyone around the world is the chicken soup to treat simple cold or flu.

Kitchen is the best place to start with when looking for a cure the natural way, it will have more than enough natural medicines to treat, at least, some common diseases/illnesses.

Chapter 1 – Herbal Medicine to Prevent and Heal Illness

Herbal medicines have been among us for centuries. Traditional folks highly recommend to use herbs instead of modern medicine as they have no side effects and many uses. Scientists are now also backing up the assumption that intake of certain herbs can reduce blood pressure and arthritis pain and they can also help with many other common as well as serious problems. Scientists are now finding out how amazingly herbs can help in killing the cells of the cancer and even help the people having drinking problems in reducing their craving for the intake of alcohol.

This chapter includes some remedies that you can add to your kitchen cabinet so that you can take full advantage of them whenever you want to, or you can add them to your cooking as well for even more benefits.

Turmeric

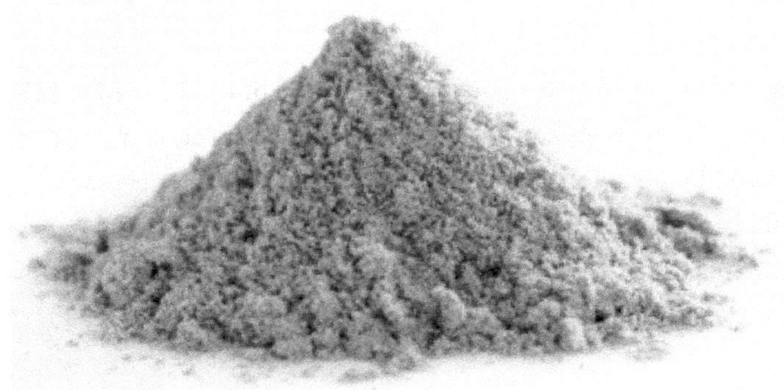

The Queen of Spices, turmeric is very common herb and has a golden color with sharp taste and has an aroma like pepper. Its use is common all over the world in cooking. It has been proven that turmeric contains many properties including anti-inflammatory, antiviral and antibacterial. Turmeric has also many other qualities, it contains Vitamin C, E and K. it is loaded with potassium and other such important proteins. Because of all these qualities, turmeric has been used for centuries to cure many diseases.

Many studies have been conducted and it has been proven that turmeric contains some active components that protects from the cancer cells and in some cases, it can destroy the cancer carrying cells completely.

Because of the anti-inflammatory properties of turmeric, it can treat osteoarthritis. Other than that, due to the antioxidant properties of turmeric, the radicals that are responsible for damaging the cells of the body are destroyed by the consumption of turmeric. By the intake of turmeric on regular basis, it has been observed that those who are suffering from rheumatoid arthritis experience relief from the mild pain and inflammation of joints.

Turmeric can also be consumed by the patients of Diabetes. It can be used to balance the insulin level. Sugar levels are also improved and the effect of medication can also be increased by taking turmeric. Other than that, turmeric can help in reducing the insulin resistance which in turns prevents the risk of getting Type 2 diabetes. Make sure to consult with the professional as turmeric with strong medication can have adverse effects.

Cinnamon

Cinnamon is a famous traditional spice and medicine as well. It has been taken from the bark of cinnamon tree and can be used in a tabular form or ground powder. It is a sweet and warm in taste and has a nice smell. It is present in many verities. The most beneficial one is essential oil of cinnamon tree's bark.

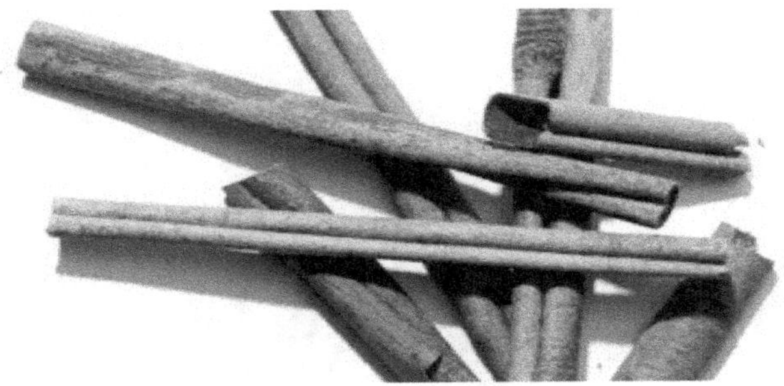

Cinnamon has properties of anti-bacterial, anti-microbial and anti-clotting along with many others. It has also many kinds of minerals that keep the body healthy and fit like iron, manganese and calcium.

Those with Type2 Diabetes can benefit from cinnamon the most, balancing their sugar level by making their body respond to insulin. One half spoon of cinnamon regularly can lower the sugar levels of blood. It is convenient to consume it as you can simply sparkle it on your meals.

It can actually boost the brain activity. By just smelling the cinnamon, the cognitive processes start working better and you are then more attentive and focused. It is also good remedy for those who have anxiety issues, smelling it soothes the brain and relaxes a person.

As cinnamon has anti-inflammatory properties, it protects the heart and the arteries that surround it from infections. Nowadays, people eat all kind of junk foods that contain fats that are unhealthy and can get clogged, all this can result in cardiovascular and other heart diseases. That's where cinnamon helps and it fights the unhealthy fats which lowers the level of cholesterol. Cinnamon also coumarin compound which thins the blood due to which blood circulation improves.

Ginger

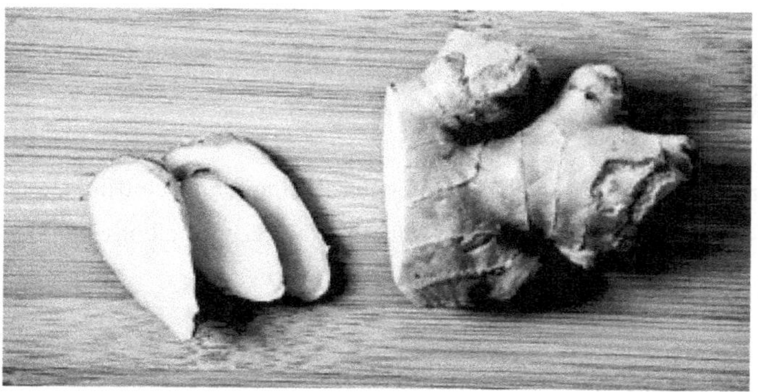

It is a known fact that ginger contains anti-bacterial, anti-fungal, anti-septic, anti-nausea and cough suppressant properties due to which it has been considered the most beneficial and inexpensive natural medicine globally. It also contains Vitamins, sodium, magnesium, potassium, iron etc. and Ginger can be used in its raw form, in its powdered form or in cooking.

Ginger helps in calming down the upset stomach; it also prevents bloating and gas by relaxing the muscles of gastrointestinal. It is also used as a cure for diarrhea and can help in improved digestion if taken after big and heavy meals.

As ginger has properties of anti-bacterial, anti-viral and anti-fungal, it can help boost your immune system and helps it fight against flu and other respiratory viruses. It also helps in relieving the fever by making your body sweat. By taking it several times a day during flu or cold, it will make the process of healing faster. It reduces menstrual pain as well by acting as pain killer because of its anti-inflammatory properties. Other than that, by drinking ginger tea, you can get a relief from migraine pain and also from the dizziness and nausea that follows.

Garlic

Garlic is usually used by people to add flavor to food but it has a key component 'allicin' that makes it a natural medicine for many illnesses as it has anti-bacterial, anti-fungal properties. Garlic also has many vitamins and nutrients. It is best to eat garlic in its raw form for better benefits as cooked garlic loses most of its medicinal properties.

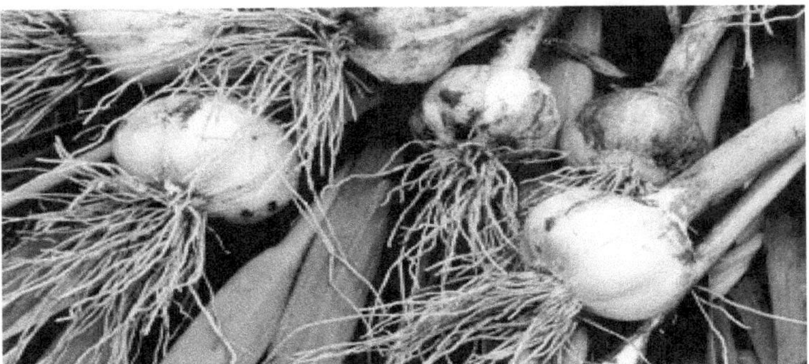

By eating 1 or 2 garlic in crushed form, you can save yourself from getting cardio-vascular diseases because it helps in the better circulation of the blood, it lowers the cholesterol and slows the arteries from getting harder. Garlic is also known to lower the blood pressure and so it is very beneficial for those who have high blood pressure. It also boosts the immune system because of the vitamins it contains and hence, helps in giving you relief in cold and flu as well.

Chapter 2 – Homemade Remedies to Treat Flu, Fever and Viral Infection

The time is here when you can have a risk of getting cold from meeting the infected person and then from cold, the symptoms might lead to flu and then from there to fever. Seasonal fever, cold and flu are thought to be spread by rhinovirus and is very contagious. The symptoms might include sore throat, stuffy nose, body aches, watery eyes, low fever and runny nose. There is no medicine that can cure flu and cold. And sometimes it is better to let the natural process do its work. There are, however, some natural remedies you can use that do not have any side effects and will give you relief and make the body's natural healing process faster and you don't even have to go out of your house.

This chapter describes the some common ingredients that can be used as natural medicine for flue, fever and cold without any side effects and these can easily be accessible.

Honey

Honey is a natural treatment to cure cold and its symptoms that include, fever, runny nose, aches etc. honey contains properties of anti-bacterial, anti-fungal which means it fights against bacteria and fungus. Honey soothes the sore and itchy throat naturally and boosts the immune system due to which it can heal the body itself faster and protects from getting the cold in future. One thing should be kept in mind that honey shouldn't be given to infants as it is too strong for them.

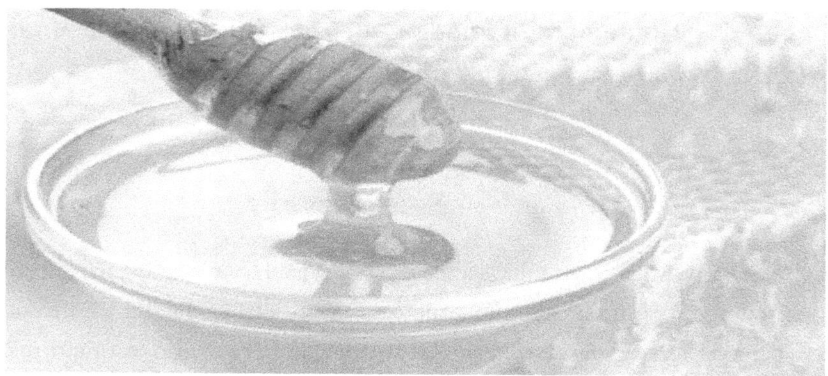

To treat fever and cold, honey could either be taken solely or in juice or tea. It can also be taken with cinnamon for better effects and you can also mix honey with two cups of warm water and after it has been cool down, gargle with it. This will soothe the throat and you will get instant relief from pain.

Cayenne Pepper

Cayenne pepper is the most convenient ingredient which can bring the fever down as it stimulates the sweat glands and makes the body temperature lower. It also helps in clearing the sinuses and respiratory passages because of its compound capsaicin.

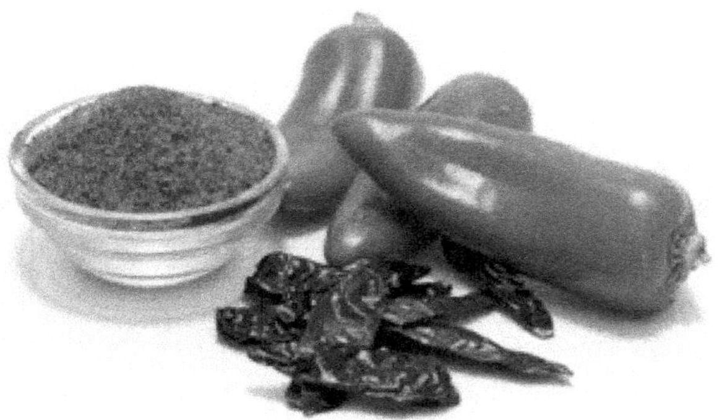

In order to consume pepper to treat the fly symptoms and fever is to mix it with a tablespoon of honey in a cup of tea. For this you can take a cup of warm water and dip a tea bag in it and a spoon full of honey and half tea spoon of cayenne pepper. Mix them all together and the drink the mixture.

Lemons and Oranges

When a person is sick, his immune system needs lots of Vitamin C and fruits like oranges and lemons are high in Vitamin C. These nutrients' loaded fruits strengthen the immune system and help it in fighting against the cold symptoms. Lemon helps in thinning the mucus, releasing the phlegm and hence, clearing the respiratory tract. Lemon if eaten raw, might not give you a pleasant feeling. Lemon remedy for flu and fever has been followed since ancient times and as they are really high in acid, they can fight off any bacteria and virus.

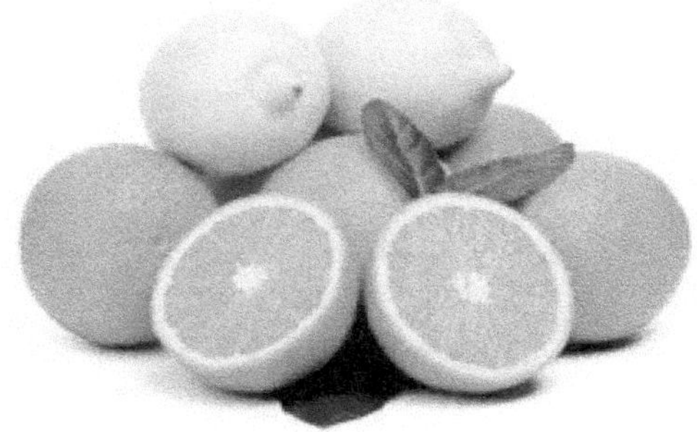

All you have to do is make a fresh juice of orange or lemon juice by mixing 1 to 2 table spoons of honey with 2 spoons of lemon juice in warm water and then drink it. Or, you can put the chopped lemon in hot water and let it settle while inhaling the steam coming from it, when the chopped lemon has been settles, mix little honey in it and drink this three to four times a day.

Eucalyptus Oil

Eucalyptus oil is made from the leaves of eucalyptus tree. The leaves are at first dried, when they are fully dried then they are being crushed and after that they are filtered so that essential oil can be extracted from them. Before using this oil as medicine, the extracted oil must be thinned. There are many vapors made of eucalyptus oil and they can stop you from coughing and in order to get the mucus out of the chest, the vapor made of this essential oil is inhaled or you can inhale the steam that has eucalyptus oil added in it. Other than that, you can put few drops on a piece of cloth and place that cloth under your pillow, this way the fumes of oil will spread during the night and helps you breathe more easily. It is also a great pain reliever, by massaging the affected area with eucalyptus oil, you will get instant relief.

Above mentioned remedies are the most common and most easy ones. There are many other ways to soothe the problems you are having because of cold or flu, but these will be most effective and most convenient. Other than that, stay warm, take warm baths and take as much rest as you can.

Chapter 3 – Remedies to Treat Headache and Body Pain

Many people, when they are suffering from pains, like headache, back pain or any other kind of pain, they will be most likely to go and take a pill. But it has been proven that pills only work 20% of the times to give relief from the pains. Other than that, painkillers have side effects and there is a possibility of making it a habit to take pills.

Person shouldn't rely on painkillers or modern medicines every time there is something of minor intensity is wrong. There are many natural and safe ways to get relief from pains. These ways have no side effects, are effective and are inexpensive and just need little effort.

There are many herbs and spices available that have medicinal properties and can act as natural medicine. Few of the exercises also come under the natural remedies. In this chapter, we will discuss few remedies that can help in relieving pain and headache.

Willow Bark

Most of the pains are due to the inflammations, to ease them people have been using willow bark from the ancient times. There is an ingredient in white willow bark which resembles the ingredient in aspirin known as the chemical salicin.

Traditional folks used to chew on the raw willow bark in order to get relief from the pains. Nowadays, these are sold as herbs that can be used to make tea. Other than that, they come as a capsule or supplement. Willow bark has many uses; it can ease the pain of head, back and many other things. Keep in mind that willow bark is only for the adult use. And it can be dangerous if used with other drugs taken to ease the pain.

Cloves

Cloves are used in variety of forms, it has been used as a spice in cooking for centuries either in its raw form or ground form. For medicine, there are clove capsules available or in its powder form. There is also clove oil available.

Cloves has many uses where there is pain concerned, toothaches, headaches and nausea, colds and many alike conditions can be eased with the help of cloves. Cloves can also be used to treat infections caused by fungus but whether it is effective or not, more studies should be conducted for that.

Clove has the natural pain reliever ingredient called eugenol. Clove oil can be rubbed on the gums to get instant relief from the toothache but only for a short while if you need to go to a dentist. If the pain is not severe, clove oil should be enough.

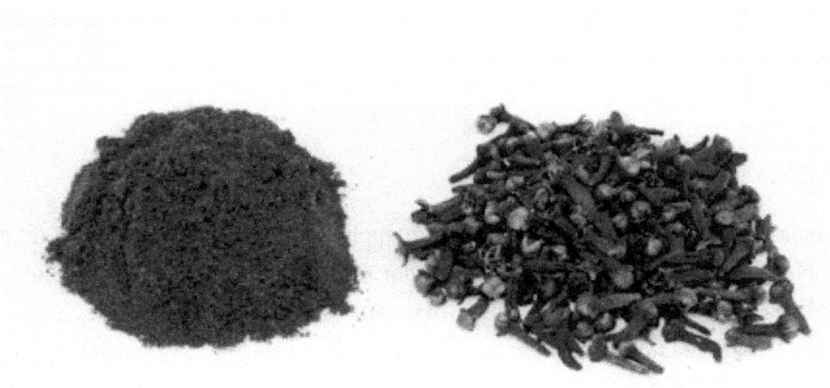

Know that, too much of a clove oil can be harmful to gums and people having bleeding disorders or who are on blood thinning medications should avoid using cloves because it might increase the bleeding.

Heat and Ice

Heat and ice are commonly used by many people as a home remedy to relieve pain instantly but sometimes, they are not as effective as they have heard they would be. That is because people are not quite aware of when should be heat and ice used. If you have a strained muscle, ligament or any tendon, it creates stiffness and swelling. The ice is firstly used to settle down the inflammation on the affected area and after it has been gone, heat should be used to decrease the stiffness.

If a person is having a headache, cold pack can reduce it to some extent. Similarly, if a person is having joint pain due to arthritis, hot water pack should be placed on the area where it pains. Hot water pack can be microwaved whenever it has to be used so it is convenient as well.

Apple Cider Vinegar

Apple Cider Vinegar has been made from apples' must. It has been proven that apple cider vinegar has many benefits from simple cold to high fever. Although there are less scientific evidences but what makes it special is its long roots in history. Traditional folks have been using apple cider vinegar as a treatment for centuries. If you are having a headache and is not settling down by itself, you can use the apple cider vinegar as a remedy.

Put one quarter spoon of apple cider vinegar in a large bowl and then pour boiling water in it till its half full. Take a towel and place it over head and all the way down so that your face is covered over the bowl with the towel. Breathe in the steam and then breathe out. Make sure your face is not too close to the bowl. Take this steam for five to ten minutes and after you are done, dry your face with the same towel and then have a drink of cool water.

Fish Oil

Fish oil is helpful in reducing migraine pains and headaches, studies suggest. It has compounds like omega-3 fatty acids due to which inflammation can be reduced and cure the blood clotting. It also lowers the blood pressure and heart beat is steadied. All of these can help in reducing the migraine pains as well because of decrease in the blood cells' inflammation that are pressing and pinching on the nerves.

You can either take 1 spoon of fish oil or there are supplements of fish oil. For the consumption of fish oil, mix 1 tablespoon of oil with one glass of fruit juice preferably orange juice and drink it up.

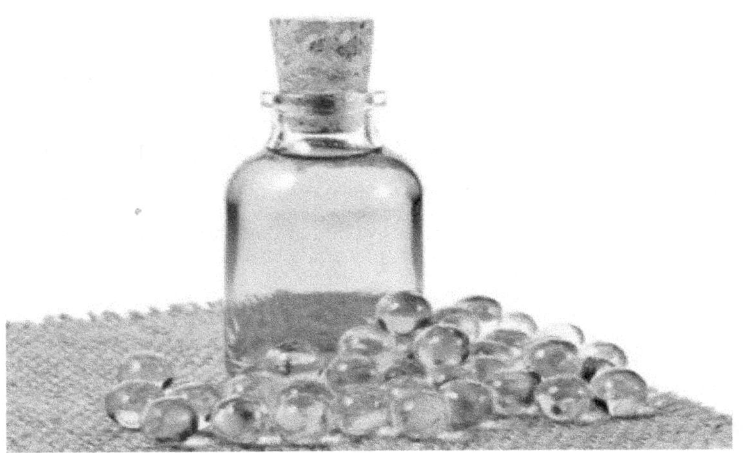

Above mentioned remedies are some of the natural ways you can heal the pain for a short period. These remedies might not work for everybody but you can try these as they have no side effects before running towards modern pharmacological solutions. Pain is the body's way of telling that there is something wrong that needs looking after. If after these remedies, the pain does not subside, check with your physician to prevent a serious issue.

Chapter 4 – Remedies for the Treatment of Throat, Nasal and Ear Infections

Ear, nose and throat are the important organs of the body and they have a connection which links them all together. If one area of these organs get infected, you will experience discomfort in all the organs. The ear and throat are linked with a tube called Eustachian tube and when there is nasal infection, the sore throat blocks this tube, due to which this tube gets swelled and as the pressure keeps on increasing in the ear, it causes pain.

This chapter includes few remedies that can ease the discomfort from throat, nasal and ear infections.

Salt

Gargling with the salt water has been effective treatment for sore throats for years and it is the best and easiest remedy.

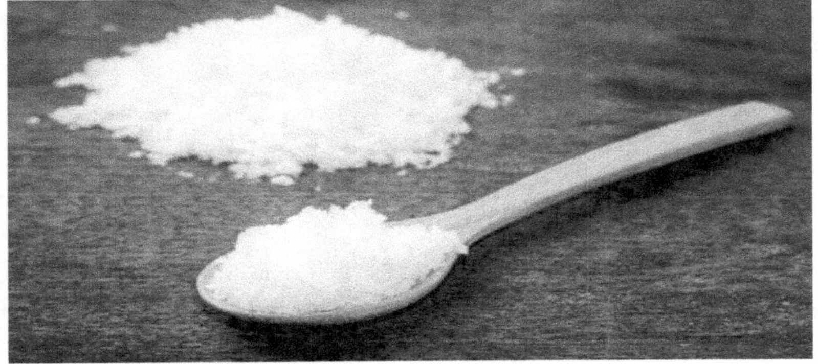

All you have to do is take one quarter spoon of salt and mix it with the hottest water that you can tolerate because gargling with cold water is ineffective. Listerine will also be effective, if you have it, mix 1 spoon of it in the salt water so that it can kill germs. Gargle with this water few times a day. Its acidic properties will help the mucus out of your system and spit out the water, do not swallow it.

Salt is also effective for the ear infections. For that, you have to heat the salt in pan and put it in the cloth, sealing its open end and when it's tolerable, put it on the ear that has been affected for 5 to 10 minutes. Try this remedy for few days. The pressure that has been inside the ear tube will be released due to the warmth of the hot salt.

Bromelain

Bromelain is found and extracted from the stem of pineapple. It basically is a protein and it is sold in the form of capsule. It has properties of anti-inflammatory due to which it is the best remedy for nasal infections as it reduces the swelling and the development of mucus in the nasal passages. It should be taken before meals, on empty stomach so that it can benefit more. Avoid using it if you are allergic to Papaya or Pineapple.

Olive Oil

Olive oil has properties of anti-inflammatory which makes it best remedy for ear infections, sore throat and congested nose. Ear infections can be caught due to the fungal or bacterial growth and development in the Eustachian tube, it could be due to anything. With the help of olive oil a person can get some relief from the blockage.

For that, heat olive oil and put few drops in the ear. This will moisten the wax and with the help of cotton sticks, remove the excess wax carefully.

If a remedy contains olive oil for cough, it gives instant relief to the itchiness due to which the cough occurs. Take one quarter lemon juice and one quarter spoon of honey and mix them. Add warm olive oil to it half cup and every hour or so, take one tablespoon of this mixture.

Basil Leaves

Basil are used to treat many kinds of illnesses like cough, nose congestion, rash, sore throat, ear infections, hives and many other conditions. It is the popular herb and those who knows its benefits usually have it grown in their gardens. It is also used in cooking. In order to get relief from ear pain and nasal infection make a tea of basil leave along with other herbs like turmeric, ginger can give you instant relief from sore throat and ear pain. You can also add little honey to it for better results. Consumption of this tea also reduces the fever symptoms.

If you are suffering just from the ear infection, you can put few drops of basil via ear dropper in the affected ear.

If you are not getting relief from these few remedies, you can always use soothers that contains eucalyptus. Try out these remedies, make sure to take a lot of rest and stay away from those who are sick and you will feel better quickly and it will probably save your trip to your physician's office.

Chapter 5 – Remedies to Treat Allergies, Cuts and Injuries

Sometimes, you get injured but the injury is minor so you don't need the feel to visit the doctor. In any case, one should not leave the cuts and injuries without any treatment as it may lead to infections. In cases of minor cuts and injuries, there are some home remedies that you can use to treat the cuts and prevent from getting infections.

Also, as the weather is changing, there are many people who are at risk of getting allergies. While some allergies could be severe and need proper attention and care of the doctor. But you can either prevent allergies to get so sever or they are minor that you can deal with them at home by using some natural home remedies having no side effects. Sometimes, even bad allergies can also be treated by the home remedies.

Red Onion Water

Onions are the best source of reducing allergies as it contains a compound called quercetin which is water soluble and that decreases the amount of body production of histamine. As onions are natural anti-histamine and Quercetin present in them, they can inhibit inflammation and open up the airways so a person can breathe easily.

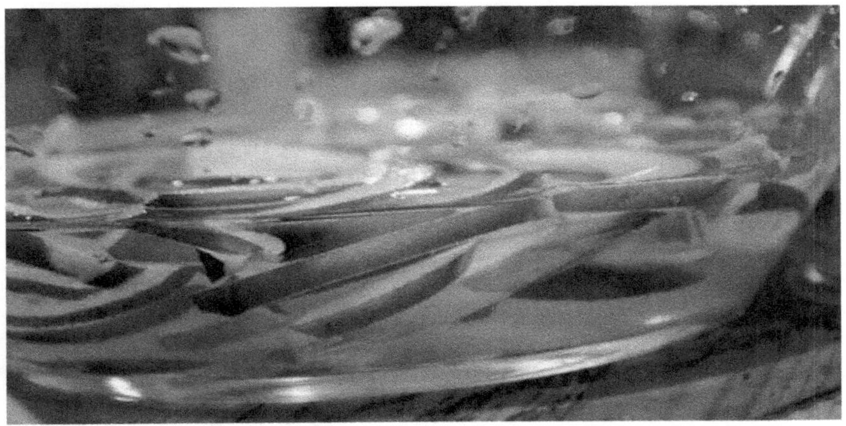

All you need to do is have one onion, 4 cups of water and honey that is raw. Slice the onion into thin layers and add these layers to water. Let them settle in the water for about 8 hours and then drink it one or two times daily. You can keep it in the fridge for four days. Every time you drink, make sure to add some honey to it.

Potato

Potatoes have the power to heal wounds and they have a quality of drawing out any kind of infection from the wounds or injuries. In order to get potato to work, make a poultice of the shredded potatoes and while changing it every 3 to 4 hours or so, keep it on the affected area the whole day. And in between changing the poultice, you should rinse the area with salt water. By doing this, inflammation will be reduced and you will be saved from infection. In order to make poultice, cut the potato and shred it. Take a cloth and place the shredded potato on it. Place it on the affected area and cover it with some material so that it can stay on the place. Leave it these for a night but make sure to remove it first thing in the morning. After you have removed the poultice, rinse it with the salt water and again cover it with the new cloth and new dressing. You should continue doing this until the wound is healed.

Aloe Vera

Aloe Vera is by far the most beneficial house plant you will find. It is used as natural remedy and as a cosmetic. It has different properties due to which it can be used to heal wounds, injuries, burns. It also improves the condition of intestine, skin, hair and many others.

Aloe Vera contains properties that make it a natural antiseptic. Because it is a natural antiseptic, it can be used in the healing process of skin tissues that are damaged, thus, it speeds up the process of recovery. In order to treat the injury or wound, first of all you have to clean the affected area thoroughly and then the pulp that has been extracted from the Aloe Vera should be applied to the wound. Take a bandage and wrap around the wound tightly and make sure that with Aloe Vera juice, bandage should be kept soaked.

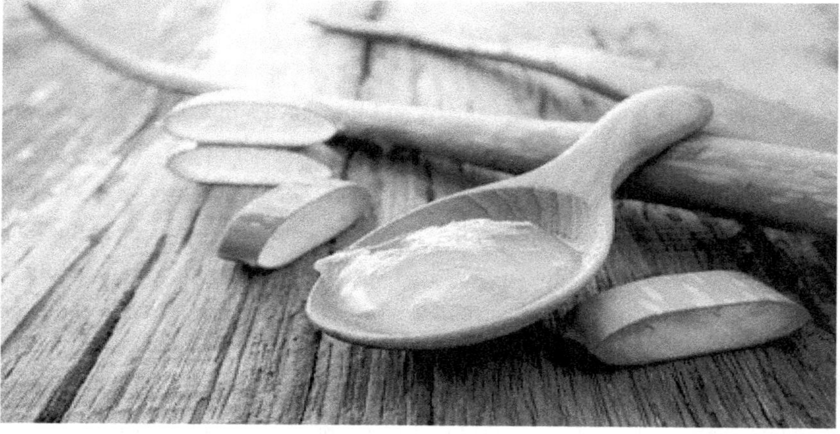

After some time, the wound should be healed and there shouldn't be any scar left. Bandage is easy to remove so you don't have to worry about any kind of pain. Aloe Vera is known to reduce different kinds of infections. Make sure to do this process during day and night until you see no scars. If there are any kind of scrapes, you can simply take aloe Leaf and scrub it over the affected area several times in the next 24 hours.

Remember, if the wounds are sever and deep, it is best to avoid using Aloe Vera. Also in the case of 3rd degree burns as it is possible that Aloe Vera will slow down the process of healing for these wounds because Aloe Vera moisturize the skin so that affects the process of wound healing as it has to be kept dry.

Conclusion

Home remedies include using vegetables, spices and herbs and for these you need not to go outside home. You can use them by just going to your kitchen. Mainly honey, garlic and ginger are the ingredients that can cure so many illnesses. From simple fevers to allergies and infections!

The best thing about home remedies is that these are without any side effects. Or even if there are any side effects they aren't long lasting and they are minor that does not even count as side effects. These natural remedies are here among us from the ancient times when there were no modern pharmacological medicines, people used to rely on these natural herbs and spices and they were much healthier than us. With the increase in modern day medication, treatment of illnesses got expensive while treating one illness causes damages to other parts of our body. People are now becoming aware of the side effects of medicine and more benefits of the natural remedies.

There are so many herbs and natural treatments out there, what this book covers are the most common and basic ones like turmeric, cinnamon, pepper and a like as healing herbs. Then there are some other remedies to treat flu, fever and cold. These include honey, eucalyptus oil, oranges and lemon and cayenne pepper.

You can also use remedies like cloves, willow bark, apple cider vinegar and fish oil for getting relief from the headaches and body pains like joint pains, back pains etc.

All in all, you can choose the easy and convenient way without any side effects and long lasting results by using natural remedies. All you have to know is your illness and what sort of remedy would work for it and you are set to go.

FREE Bonus Reminder

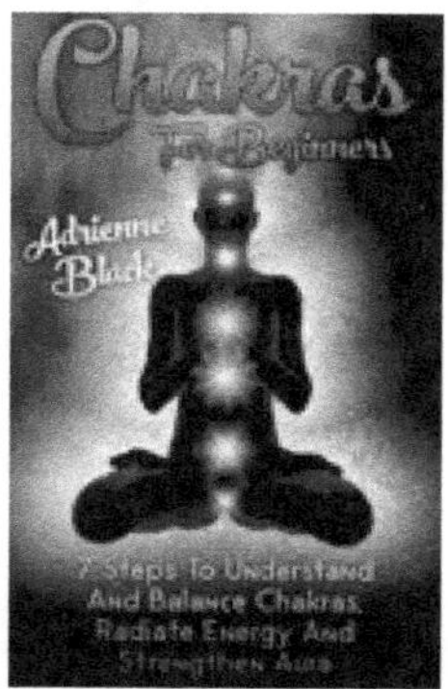

If you have not grabbed it yet, please go ahead and download your special bonus E book *"Chakras for Beginners. 7 Steps To Understand And Balance Chakras, Radiate Energy, And Strengthen Aura"*.

Simply Click the Button Below

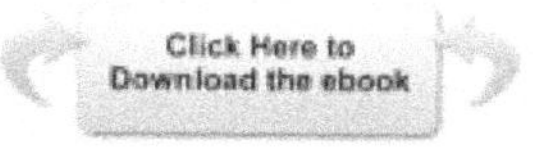

OR Go to This Page

http://lifehacksworld.com/free

BONUS #2: More Free & Discounted Books & Products

Do you want to receive more Free/Discounted Books or Products?

We have a mailing list where we send out our new Books or Products when they go free or with a discount on Amazon. Click on the link below to sign up for Free & Discount Book & Product Promotions.

=> Sign Up for Free & Discount Book & Product Promotions <=

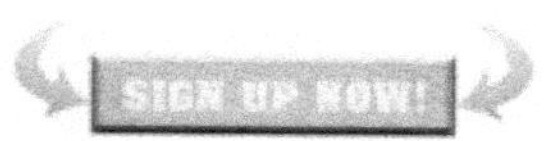

OR Go to this URL

http://zbit.ly/1WBb1Ek